This Notebook Belongs To:

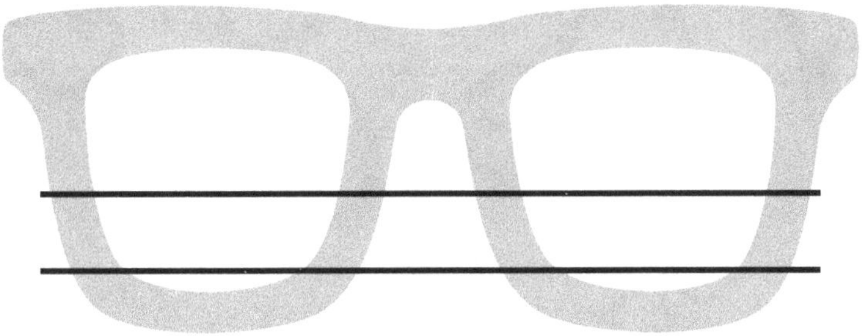

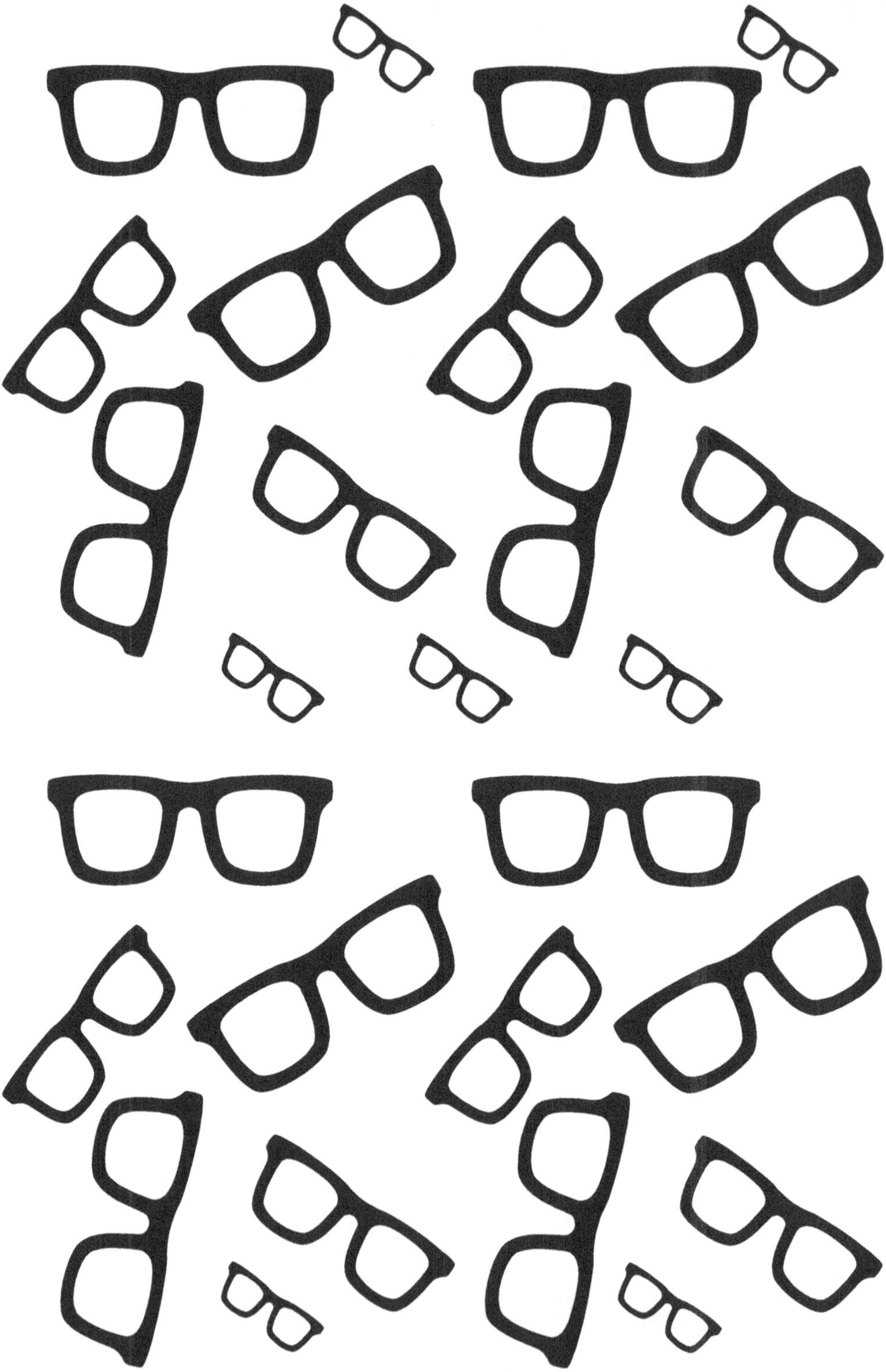

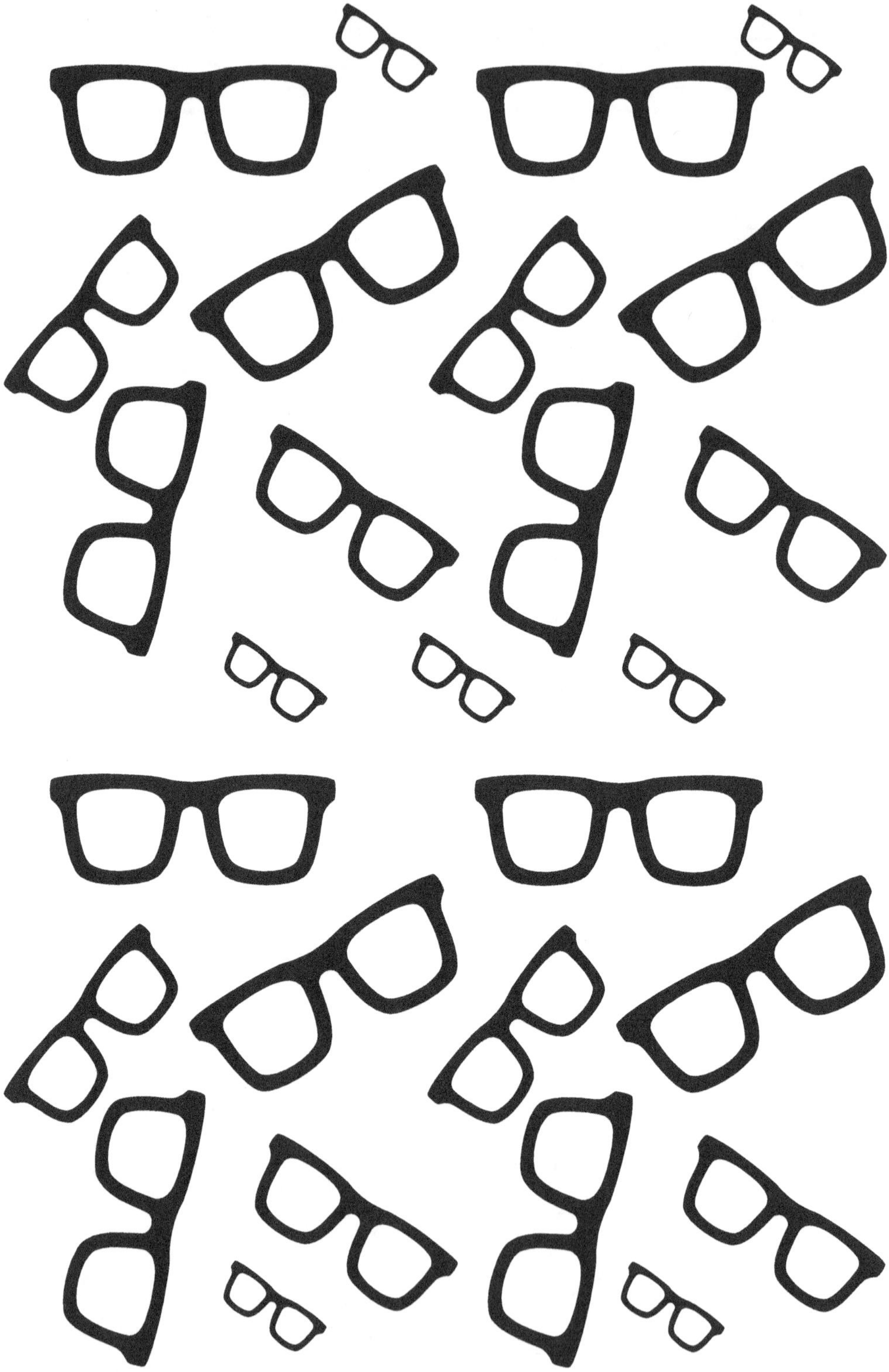

www.ingramcontent.com/pod-product-compliance
Lightning Source LLC
Chambersburg PA
CBHW070652220526
45466CB00001B/410
9781676999270